PLATELET-RICH PLASMA THERAPY FOR BEGINNERS

Comprehensive Guide To Understanding Treatments, Benefits, Applications, And Techniques For Effective Healing And Regeneration

DR SAWYER DIEGO

DISCLAMER

Nothing in this book should be interpreted as medical advice; it is meant exclusively for educational reasons. Regarding their specific health issues and treatment options, readers are urged to speak with licensed healthcare professionals. The publisher and author disclaim all liability for any errors or omissions in the material provided, as well as for any negative effects that may arise from using or abusing the information. Although every attempt has been taken to guarantee that the material in this book is correct as of the date of publishing, new research may have superseded some of the content because medical knowledge is always changing. It is recommended that readers confirm the most recent medical recommendations and guidelines. The reader of this book undertakes to release the author and publisher from any claims or liabilities resulting from the use of this information, and understands and accepts the inherent risks connected with healthcare decisions.

TABLE OF CONTENTS

ABOUT THE BOOK

"Platelet-Rich Plasma (PRP) Therapy for Beginners" is an essential resource for anyone wishing to learn about and investigate the cutting-edge treatment alternatives provided by PRP therapy. It explores the principles, advantages, and real-world uses of PRP therapy, making it understandable to medical professionals as well as patients who are interested in its potential.

In the first section of the book, Platelet-Rich Plasma (PRP) is defined, its constituent parts are explained, and the history, development, and evolution of PRP in the medical and aesthetic domains are thoroughly covered. Readers are also given an understanding of the various uses of PRP therapy, from orthopedic ailments like tendinitis and joint injuries to dermatological applications like treating hair loss and facial rejuvenation. PRP's applications in dentistry and oral health, chronic pain management, and new research domains are also covered, emphasizing the adaptability of PRP in contemporary medicine.

The process of getting ready for PRP therapy is one of the most important topics that is thoroughly discussed. It stresses the value of pre-procedure guidelines, initial consultations, and comprehension of the possible risks and benefits. It also covers insurance coverage and financial concerns so that potential patients can make well-informed decisions.

After that, the book goes into great detail about the actual PRP therapy process, taking readers through each step of blood sample extraction, laboratory processing, injection techniques, and post-procedure care. Clinical studies, patient testimonials, and comparisons with alternative treatments all support the importance of monitoring progress and controlling expectations regarding treatment outcomes.

Integration of PRP therapy with other treatments, such as physical therapy or surgical procedures, is explored to maximize therapeutic outcomes in multidisciplinary healthcare settings. Safety considerations are paramount, with a thorough discussion on common side effects, managing discomfort, and minimizing risks through proper preparation and medical oversight.

After PRP therapy, recovery, and rehabilitation are also covered; this includes the anticipated time frame, physical activity limitations, rehabilitation exercises, dietary suggestions, and the continuous monitoring needed for the best possible outcome. Financial aspects, such as cost considerations, insurance coverage, legal considerations, and patient rights, are fully described to help readers navigate the practical aspects of treatment.

The book addresses frequently asked questions (FAQs) and common concerns raised by patients regarding pain, sustainability of treatment, frequency of sessions, and the educational empowerment required to make informed healthcare decisions.

CHAPTER ONE

PLATELET-RICH PLASMA THERAPY OVERVIEW

WHAT IS PRP, OR PLATELET-RICH PLASMA?

A small sample of your blood is drawn, usually from your arm, and then placed in a centrifuge, which spins the blood at high speeds to separate the platelets from other blood components. The resulting plasma is rich in a higher concentration of platelets than usual, hence the name "platelet-rich plasma." Platelet-rich plasma (PRP) therapy is a medical treatment that uses the natural healing power of platelets found in your blood to promote tissue repair and regeneration.

PRP is prepared and then injected directly into the area that needs to be treated. This concentrated form of platelets contains proteins and growth factors that are essential for healing injuries and promoting tissue regeneration.

Sports medicine, orthopedics, dermatology, and other medical specialties frequently employ PRP therapy to relieve pain and speed healing from conditions like osteoarthritis, chronic wounds, and tendon injuries.

Although PRP therapy is safe because it uses the patient's blood, which lowers the risk of allergic reactions or rejection, the degree of discomfort experienced by patients during the procedure—which is carried out in a medical office setting—varies depending on the particular condition being treated and individual health factors.

 PRP is still a subject of active research and development, with ongoing studies examining its potential applications and refining treatment protocols for optimal results.

PRP THERAPY'S ADVANTAGES

PRP therapy stimulates the body's natural healing processes, which can lead to improved outcomes in conditions like tendonitis, ligament injuries, and joint pain. One of the main benefits of PRP therapy is that it can speed up tissue repair and promote faster healing times than traditional methods. PRP therapy works by directly applying a concentrated dose of growth factors to the site of inflammation or injury.

The minimally invasive nature of PRP therapy is another important advantage. Unlike surgical procedures, PRP injections are done in a doctor's office, resulting in little recovery time or discomfort for the patient.

This outpatient treatment option allows people to return to their regular activities soon after the procedure, which makes it a convenient option for people with hectic schedules or demanding jobs.

Since PRP therapy uses the patient's blood components, there is less chance of allergic reactions or rejection, which makes it a safe and effective treatment option for people who might not be candidates for surgery or who would prefer non-surgical interventions for their medical conditions.

Additionally, **PRP** therapy is frequently preferred due to its low risk of adverse reactions or complications.

SECURITY AND ADVERSE REACTIONS

Since **PRP** uses the patient's blood, there is a much lower chance of disease transmission or allergic reactions; however, as with any medical procedure, there are possible side effects and risks to take into account. PRP therapy is generally regarded as safe when performed by qualified healthcare professionals.

In rare instances, patients may experience injection site infection; however, strict sterile techniques help minimize this risk. Common side effects of PRP therapy include mild pain, swelling, or bruising at the injection site. These symptoms are usually transient and resolve on their own within a few days.

Patients who are thinking about PRP therapy should speak with their healthcare provider about any conditions they currently have as well as their medical history. This will help guarantee that PRP is a suitable course of treatment and enable the provider to address any concerns about possible side effects or complications. Patients can improve the safety and efficacy of PRP therapy for their unique medical needs by adhering to recommended guidelines and receiving treatment from qualified professionals.

THE OPERATION OF PRP THERAPY

During the PRP procedure, a small sample of the patient's blood is drawn and processed in a centrifuge to concentrate these platelets. Platelets are tiny cells in the blood that contain proteins called growth factors, responsible for initiating tissue repair and regeneration.

PRP therapy works by harnessing the healing properties of platelets, which play a crucial role in the body's natural healing process.

The high concentration of growth factors in platelet-rich plasma (PRP) stimulates the formation of new collagen, blood vessels, and connective tissue, which is necessary for repairing damaged tissues and reducing inflammation. This regenerative process helps accelerate healing and alleviate symptoms associated with various musculoskeletal and dermatological conditions. Once the PRP is prepared, it can be administered directly through injection to the injured or affected area.

PRP therapy is dependent upon several factors, such as the particular ailment being addressed, the patient's general health, and compliance with aftercare instructions.

It may be necessary to undergo multiple PRP sessions to achieve the best possible outcome, especially in cases of chronic conditions or injuries that need to be continuously managed. As research advances, medical professionals adjust PRP treatment regimens to optimize the therapeutic benefits and enhance patient outcomes.

WHY TAKE A LOOK AT PRP THERAPY?

For those looking for non-surgical treatments for joint pain, musculoskeletal injuries, and dermatological conditions, PRP therapy is a compelling option. One of the main benefits of PRP therapy is that it can stimulate natural healing processes in place of invasive surgery, which lowers the risks involved with the procedure and expedites patient recovery.

For athletes and active people, PRP therapy may offer an advantage in recovering from sports-related injuries and regaining peak performance levels. Additionally, PRP therapy can be customized to target specific areas of concern, delivering concentrated growth factors directly to the site of injury or inflammation. This targeted approach enhances the effectiveness of treatment and promotes faster healing compared to traditional methods alone.

PRP has proven effective in treating a wide range of conditions, including osteoarthritis, tendonitis, chronic wounds, and hair loss. Its versatility across medical specialties further supports its potential as a valuable therapeutic tool in modern medicine, providing patients with individualized treatment options that are in line with their healthcare goals and lifestyle preferences.

CHAPTER TWO

AN OVERVIEW OF PLATELET-RICH PLASMA (PRP) TREATMENT

PRP: DEFINITION AND CONSTITUENTS

A small sample of the patient's blood is processed to concentrate the platelets, which are essential components of blood known for their role in clotting and wound healing. In PRP therapy, the concentrated platelets are injected into the target area, where they release growth factors that stimulate tissue regeneration and repair. Because of its potential to enhance healing processes naturally, platelet-rich plasma (PRP) therapy is a medical treatment that uses the patient's blood to promote healing in various conditions.

Plasma, the liquid portion of blood, acts as a medium for transporting platelets and growth factors to the injured tissues. During PRP preparation, the blood sample is centrifuged to separate these components and concentrate the platelets, which are then carefully injected into the affected area. Platelets contain bioactive proteins, such as transforming growth factor beta (TGF-β), platelet-derived growth factor (PDGF), and vascular endothelial growth factor (VEGF), which play key roles in tissue repair and regeneration.

Since its inception in the 1970s, PRP therapy has had a significant evolution in both medical and aesthetic fields. Originally used for maxillofacial surgery to promote bone healing, PRP has expanded into orthopedics to treat tendon injuries like tennis elbow and knee osteoarthritis, dermatology to rejuvenate skin and hair growth, and dentistry to promote healing after dental procedures.

THE DEVELOPMENT AND HISTORY OF PRP THERAPY

The concept of using platelets for therapeutic purposes dates back to the 1970s when PRP was first used in maxillofacial surgery to aid in bone regeneration.

Over the years, advances in biotechnology and medical research have refined the preparation and application of PRP, expanding its use across various medical disciplines. Platelet-rich plasma (PRP) therapy has a rich history rooted in medical research and innovation.

There have been several notable turning points in the development of PRP therapy. First, in sports medicine, PRP was used to treat sports-related injuries in athletes, like tendonitis and ligament injuries. It was also preferred in orthopedic practices because it sped up healing and shortened recovery times. Later, as research progressed, PRP was used in aesthetic medicine for skin rejuvenation, wound healing, and hair restoration procedures.

PRP therapy is still evolving today due to ongoing clinical studies and technological advancements. Its non-surgical approach, minimal side effects, and use of autologous (patient-derived) components have all contributed to its growing acceptance and integration into mainstream medical treatments worldwide.

UTILIZATIONS IN THE DOMAINS OF MEDICINE AND BEAUTY

With its regenerative properties stimulating tissue repair and reducing inflammation, platelet-rich plasma (PRP) therapy is a versatile treatment option for a variety of conditions with broad applications in both the medical and aesthetic fields. In the medical domain, PRP is widely used in orthopedics to accelerate healing in musculoskeletal injuries like tendonitis, ligament sprains, and osteoarthritis.

For skin rejuvenation treatments, PRP is injected or applied topically to stimulate collagen production, improve skin texture, and reduce fine lines and wrinkles. For hair restoration, PRP injections into the scalp help stimulate dormant hair follicles, increase hair thickness, and slow down hair loss, providing a non-invasive alternative to traditional hair transplant procedures. PRP is well-known in dermatology and aesthetic medicine for its ability to rejuvenate skin and promote hair growth.

PRP therapy is not only used for musculoskeletal and cosmetic purposes; it is also used in dentistry to improve bone graft healing and tissue regeneration after oral surgeries. Because of its inherent healing qualities and low risk of side effects, PRP therapy is a preferred adjunct therapy for dental implant procedures and periodontal treatments. As new research reveals even more potential uses, PRP therapy stays at the forefront of regenerative medicine, constantly broadening its scope in clinical practice.

HEALING'S MECHANISM OF ACTION

Platelets, rich in growth factors such as transforming growth factor beta (TGF-β), vascular endothelial growth factor (VEGF), and platelet-derived growth factor (PDGF), play a crucial role in tissue repair and regeneration. When injected into injured tissues, PRP releases these growth factors, which stimulate cellular proliferation, angiogenesis (formation of new blood vessels), and matrix synthesis.

This is the basis for the mechanism of action of Platelet-Rich Plasma (PRP) therapy.

The concentrated platelets in PRP also function as a reservoir of cytokines and chemokines that modulate the immune response, further supporting the healing process without inducing adverse immune reactions. Upon injection, PRP activates local stem cells and fibroblasts, promoting collagen formation and tissue remodeling. This process enhances the healing response by accelerating the repair of damaged tissues, reducing inflammation, and improving overall tissue function.

PRP therapy has been shown to have therapeutic effects in conditions where traditional treatments have not been as effective or have required longer recovery times. PRP injections into tendons or joint tissues in orthopedics have been shown to improve healing in chronic injuries and degenerative conditions like osteoarthritis. PRP's regenerative properties have improved skin texture and tone in dermatology, where it is being used to treat aging skin, scars, and alopecia. PRP therapy is still a promising therapy as research into its mechanisms is ongoing.

DIFFERENCES IN PRP PREPARATION METHODS

Platelet-rich plasma (PRP) therapy comprises a range of preparation methods that are specifically designed to maximize the concentration and bioactivity of platelets for particular therapeutic applications. The most widely utilized PRP preparation methods are leukocyte-rich PRP (L-PRP), double-spin centrifugation, and single-spin centrifugation; each has unique benefits based on the specific clinical situation and treatment objectives.

Double-spin centrifugation, on the other hand, involves two rounds of centrifugation to achieve higher platelet concentrations and purity. This method is preferred in complex orthopedic cases and advanced aesthetic treatments requiring precise control over platelet concentration and bioactive factors. Single-spin centrifugation is a basic PRP preparation technique that involves a single round of centrifugation to separate blood components. This technique yields a moderate concentration of platelets suspended in plasma, suitable for general orthopedic applications and basic aesthetic procedures.

Compared to standard platelet-rich plasma (PRP), leukocyte-rich PRP (L-PRP) contains a higher concentration of leukocytes (white blood cells), which are white blood cells that contribute to the immune response and may improve tissue healing through additional growth factors and cytokines. L-PRP is frequently used in chronic tendon injuries, where tissue degeneration and inflammation are prominent, to effectively modulate the inflammatory environment and promote tissue regeneration.

CHAPTER THREE

MEDICAL CONDITIONS PRP THERAPY TREATS

CONDITIONS RELATED TO ORTHOPEDICS

To accelerate tissue repair and improve joint function over time, Platelet-Rich Plasma (PRP) therapy has become more and more popular as a treatment for a variety of orthopedic conditions, including tendonitis and joint injuries. PRP is injected directly into the affected joint to promote healing and reduce inflammation. The process starts with a small blood sample from the patient, usually from the arm, which is then processed to concentrate the platelets. These platelets, rich in growth factors and proteins, are then injected back into the injured joint under ultrasound guidance.

PRP therapy treats tendons that are inflamed or degenerate. As with joint injuries, blood is drawn, and processed to separate the platelets, and the concentrated PRP is injected into the tendon.

The growth factors that are released from the platelets promote tendon healing and regeneration, reducing pain and enhancing tendon strength. Depending on the severity of the condition and each patient's response, a series of PRP injections may be administered.

PRP therapy for orthopedic conditions is a viable option for patients who prefer non-surgical treatments or who have not responded to conventional therapies. It functions as a minimally invasive alternative for patients seeking relief from joint pain and tendon issues. It also plays a role in enhancing natural healing processes without invasive surgery.

CONDITIONS RELATED TO DERMATOLOGY

In the context of hair loss, platelet-rich plasma (PRP) is prepared by extracting blood from the patient and processing it to isolate the plasma. This rich in growth factors is then injected into the scalp, targeting areas affected by hair thinning or baldness.

Throughout multiple treatment sessions, the growth factors stimulate hair follicles, promoting hair growth and improving hair density. Platelet-rich plasma (PRP) therapy has shown promising results in dermatology, particularly in treating conditions like hair loss and facial rejuvenation.

Using the patient's platelets, PRP facial rejuvenation improves skin tone and texture. PRP is extracted from blood and separated into plasma; it is then either injected into targeted facial areas or applied topically during microneedling procedures. PRP's growth factors stimulate collagen production and improve blood flow, which results in smoother, firmer skin and a reduction in the appearance of fine lines and wrinkles.

The use of PRP in dermatology highlights its function in natural skin and hair rejuvenation, providing patients with non-surgical options and little recovery time. PRP therapy is a popular treatment in cosmetic dermatology because it uses the body's healing mechanisms to effectively address aesthetic concerns.

APPLICATIONS IN DENTISTRY AND ORAL HEALTH

Dental implant surgery is one common procedure where Platelet-Rich Plasma (PRP) therapy is used because of its regenerative properties; PRP is prepared from the patient's blood and applied directly to the surgical site to promote faster healing and lower the risk of complications. PRP is applied to the implant site to enhance bone regeneration and integration of the implant.

PRP's growth factors support tissue regeneration and repair, which helps the healing process following periodontal treatments or oral surgeries. The concentrated platelets help to accelerate wound closure and reduce inflammation, improving overall oral health outcomes. Gum disease and oral ulcers are other areas where PRP is beneficial.

Dental professionals can enhance healing processes and improve patient satisfaction with less post-operative discomfort and faster recovery times by utilizing the patient's blood components. PRP's integration into dental practice highlights its potential to optimize treatment outcomes through natural healing mechanisms.

MANAGEMENT OF CHRONIC PAIN

With its concentrated growth factors, platelet-rich plasma (PRP) therapy has become a promising treatment modality for chronic pain management, especially in musculoskeletal conditions and soft tissue injuries. PRP injections are given directly into the affected area for conditions such as arthritis-related pain or chronic tendon injuries. PRP therapy targets the underlying causes of discomfort and promotes tissue repair and inflammation reduction.

PRP injections are intended to strengthen and promote healing in chronic tendon injuries, such as tennis elbow or Achilles tendinopathy. The process entails drawing blood from the patient, separating the PRP, and then injecting the PRP under ultrasound guidance into the injured tendon. By injecting the

PRP precisely where it is needed, this targeted approach can potentially minimize the need for lengthy medication regimens or invasive surgical procedures.

PRP's application in the treatment of chronic pain highlights both its non-surgical nature and its potential to offer patients with persistent musculoskeletal pain long-lasting relief. By utilizing the body's natural healing factors, PRP presents a viable adjunctive therapy or alternative to traditional pain management techniques.

NEW FIELDS OF STUDY

In addition to its well-established uses, Platelet-Rich Plasma (PRP) therapy is being investigated for its potential in several rapidly developing fields of research. One such field is regenerative medicine, where the potential of PRP to stimulate tissue repair and regeneration is being investigated for conditions such as osteoarthritis and spinal disc degeneration. PRP's ability to modulate inflammation and stimulate cartilage regeneration is being studied to create more effective treatments for these difficult-to-treat conditions.

Preliminary research suggests that PRP may help protect brain tissue, reduce inflammation, and support recovery mechanisms following neurological insults.

Ongoing research aims to elucidate the mechanisms behind these effects and optimize PRP protocols for clinical application. Another emerging area of study is PRP's neuroprotective effects in neurological disorders, such as stroke and traumatic brain injury.

PRP therapy is being researched further in the field of sports medicine because it may help athletes recover more quickly from sports-related injuries like ligament tears and muscle strains.

It can also minimize the chance of recurrent injuries by improving tissue repair and minimizing athletes' recovery time.

Further research into PRP therapy's mechanisms of action and clinical applications holds promise for expanding its use across various medical specialties and possibly improving outcomes for patients facing complex health challenges. These emerging research areas highlight PRP therapy's versatility and ongoing evolution as a therapeutic modality.

CHAPTER FOUR

GETTING READY FOR PRP TREATMENT

FIRST MEETING WITH A MEDICAL PROFESSIONAL

The first step in getting ready for PRP therapy is making an appointment with a dermatologist or regenerative medicine specialist. In this important consultation, the doctor will examine your medical history and current condition to determine whether PRP therapy is right for you. They will also talk about your goals for PRP therapy, such as skin rejuvenation, hair restoration, or another application.

During the consultation, your provider will answer any questions or concerns you may have about the procedure and make sure you know exactly what to expect. They will also evaluate your expectations and talk about realistic outcomes based on your unique circumstances and the intended goals of the treatment.

The PRP procedure includes explaining in detail how platelet-rich plasma is extracted from your blood, processed, and then injected into the treatment area.

Following your initial appointment, if you and your healthcare practitioner determine that PRP therapy is a good fit, you'll go on to the next stages, which involve getting ready for the procedure and following all rules to maximize safety and effectiveness.

PRE-PROCEDURE INSTRUCTIONS AND LIMITATIONS

To optimize the benefits of PRP therapy and reduce risks, there are a few rules and restrictions that must be followed before the procedure. Your healthcare provider will provide you with specific instructions based on your needs. '

These rules usually include avoiding drugs and supplements that can alter platelet function or raise the risk of bleeding, such as blood thinners and non-steroidal anti-inflammatory drugs (NSAIDs).

In the days preceding your PRP treatment, your physician may also recommend that you abstain from smoking and alcohol consumption because these substances can impair circulation and promote general healing. It is also important to stay properly hydrated to guarantee the best possible blood flow and platelet function during the procedure.

In addition, it is important to mentally and emotionally prepare yourself for PRP therapy. You can lower anxiety and manage expectations by being aware of the treatment's limitations and potential outcomes. By following these pre-procedure guidelines and restrictions, you can increase the efficacy of PRP therapy and facilitate a more seamless recovery process.

RECOGNIZING POTENTIAL BENEFITS AND RISKS

PRP therapy, like any medical procedure, has potential risks and benefits that should be fully understood before proceeding.

The main advantage of PRP therapy is that, depending on the area being treated, concentrated platelets are thought to stimulate tissue repair, collagen production, and hair follicle growth.

PRP therapy does carry some risks, though, which you should be aware of. These risks include minor pain or discomfort at the injection site, temporary swelling, bruising, or infection; rarer side effects include allergic reactions to the injected plasma or nerve injury; your healthcare provider will go over all of these risks in detail during your consultation and offer suggestions to reduce them.

You can make an educated decision about pursuing PRP therapy by weighing the potential risks against the expected benefits and speaking with your healthcare provider. Results may vary depending on individual factors such as age, general health, and the specific condition being treated. Some patients may notice improvements after a single session, while others may require multiple treatments to achieve desired outcomes.

EXPECTATIONS AND MENTAL PREPARATION

Understanding the goal of PRP therapy, possible side effects, and the recuperation period is essential to psychologically and emotionally preparing for the surgery. It's common to experience mixed emotions when undergoing any kind of medical procedure, particularly one that aims to improve one's beauty or health.

Your healthcare provider will discuss realistic outcomes based on your unique condition and treatment goals. This discussion helps you align your expectations with what PRP therapy can realistically achieve. While PRP therapy offers promising results for many patients, individual responses can vary.

Mental preparation also includes getting ready for the physical side of the process, such as anticipating any pain during and after the injections; your provider might suggest ways to deal with pain or discomfort, like using cold packs or taking small amounts of medication as needed.

You can approach PRP therapy with confidence and maximize your experience and results by being aware of the process, establishing reasonable expectations, and psychologically preparing for it.

INSURANCE COVERAGE AND FINANCIAL CONSIDERATIONS

Financial considerations should be made before beginning PRP therapy because the cost of the procedure can vary based on the provider, location, and particular treatment area.

PRP therapy is usually paid for out of pocket because it is regarded as an elective procedure and may not be covered by health insurance plans.

Some healthcare facilities provide financing alternatives or payment plans to help manage upfront expenses; during your initial consultation, address the overall cost of PRP therapy, including any additional fees for consultations, follow-up sessions, or essential pre-procedure diagnostics.

It's also a good idea to inquire about your health insurance provider's coverage of PRP therapy. While many insurers do not pay for cosmetic procedures that can be done electively, some may pay a portion of the cost if PRP therapy is deemed medically necessary for a specific injury or condition.

You can make well-informed judgments about pursuing PRP therapy and set aside money for the procedure and associated costs by carefully weighing the financial ramifications and looking into payment options.

CHAPTER FIVE

THE PROCESS OF PRP THERAPY

PROCEDURE FOR PRP EXTRACTION IN DETAIL

A small amount of your blood is drawn, usually from your arm, just like in a routine blood test. The collected blood is then placed into a specialized centrifuge machine, which spins rapidly to separate its components based on their densities.

The heavier red blood cells settle at the bottom of this centrifugation process, while the lighter plasma and platelets concentrate at the top. This meticulous extraction process is the first step in the process of using platelet-rich plasma (PRP) therapy.

The separated plasma is then carefully extracted from the tube, containing a high concentration of platelets; further processing is then applied to this plasma to guarantee that it contains the ideal concentration of platelets and growth factors that are advantageous for the intended therapy; all of this is done under sterile conditions to prevent contamination and guarantee the purity of the PRP solution.

This extraction approach guarantees that the PRP is rich in platelets and growth factors, which are crucial for stimulating tissue repair and regeneration when supplied to the targeted location. Lastly, after the PRP solution is created, it is ready for immediate use in the therapeutic procedure.

PROCESSING OF A BLOOD SAMPLE IN A LABORATORY

The blood sample is obtained for platelet-rich plasma therapy, and then it is carefully processed in the lab to separate the platelet-rich plasma. The blood is initially placed into tubes designed to keep the components intact throughout transportation to the lab and to prevent clotting.

Once in the lab, the tubes go through a crucial process called centrifugation, which divides the blood into its constituent parts according to densities.

The centrifuge spins the tubes quickly, causing the platelets-containing plasma to rise to the top layer of the tube and the heavier red blood cells to settle at the bottom.

To ensure that the final PRP solution is optimized for therapeutic use, quality control measures are implemented throughout the processing to maintain the purity and efficacy of the PRP solution before it is administered to the patient. After centrifugation, the plasma layer is carefully extracted using sterile techniques to prevent contamination.

METHODS OF INJECTION AND ADMINISTRATION

PRP therapy is administered using exact injection techniques that ensure the concentrated platelet-rich plasma is delivered to the intended area efficiently. The treatment area is thoroughly cleaned before the injection to minimize the chance of infection. The doctor determines the exact injection sites based on clinical evaluation and diagnostic imaging if needed, to treat a particular condition, such as hair loss or joint pain.

The prepared PRP solution is injected directly into the identified area or areas that require treatment using a fine needle. The injection procedure is usually quick and minimally invasive, aimed at delivering the PRP solution precisely where it can exert its therapeutic effects. Anesthesia is not necessary, though patients may feel some mild discomfort during the injection.

Assuring that the PRP solution reaches its intended target effectively and promotes tissue repair and regeneration at the site of injury or concern is the aim of the injection technique.

Following the PRP injection, the doctor may apply a bandage or provide specific post-injection instructions, such as avoiding strenuous activities or applying ice to reduce swelling.

AFTER-PROCEDURE MONITORING AND ASSISTANCE

To maximize recovery and maximize the therapeutic benefits of PRP therapy, patients are usually instructed to rest and refrain from strenuous activities for a predetermined amount of time after the procedure. Depending on the area that was treated, additional post-procedure instructions may include using ice packs to minimize swelling, avoiding extreme heat or sunlight, and taking prescribed medications if needed.

The treating physician schedules follow-up appointments regularly to monitor the patient's progress and evaluate the patient's response to PRP therapy.

In these follow-up visits, the physician reviews any potential side effects or complications, assesses whether the patient's symptoms have improved, and modifies the treatment plan as necessary based on the patient's unique response.

The attainment of optimal results from PRP therapy is contingent upon patient compliance with post-procedure care instructions. Patients who diligently adhere to these instructions can facilitate the healing process and optimize the long-term advantages of treatment, thereby fostering tissue repair and regeneration in the treated region.

TRACKING DEVELOPMENT AND ANTICIPATED OUTCOMES

PRP therapy requires continuous evaluation and communication between the patient and the healthcare provider to track progress and evaluate expected outcomes. Depending on the condition being treated, patients may experience some immediate improvements in the first few weeks after treatment, such as decreased pain or increased hair growth.

The doctor keeps an eye on the patient's progress over the next few weeks and months by scheduling follow-up appointments.

In these visits, the doctor assesses the patient's response to PRP therapy, taking into account variables like pain intensity, range of motion, thickness of hair, or other pertinent indicators specific to the treated area.

Anticipated outcomes from platelet-rich plasma (PRP) therapy are contingent upon the patient's health status, the severity of the condition, and the particular treatment objectives.

While some patients may show improvement over time, others may need several PRP sessions to attain the best results. The healthcare provider collaborates closely with the patient to modify the treatment plan as needed, guaranteeing individualized attention and optimizing the therapeutic benefits of platelet-rich plasma.

Regular assessments and plan modifications help to optimize outcomes and promote long-term healing and tissue regeneration.

Patients can actively participate in their treatment journey and achieve the best possible results from PRP therapy by keeping track of their progress and keeping lines of communication open with the healthcare provider.

CHAPTER SIX

ADVANTAGES AND PERFORMANCE OF PRP THERAPY

RESEARCH FINDINGS AND CLINICAL STUDIES

PRP therapy, which involves isolating and concentrating platelets from the patient's blood and injecting them into the target area, has gained a lot of attention recently due to its potential therapeutic benefits across a variety of medical fields.

Clinical studies and research findings consistently highlight PRP therapy's efficacy in promoting tissue repair and regeneration. PRP therapy accelerates healing processes by stimulating cellular repair mechanisms and reducing pain. PRP therapy is particularly effective in orthopedic conditions like tendon injuries, osteoarthritis, and muscle strains. For example, studies have shown that PRP injections can reduce pain and improve function in patients with chronic tendon pr

Further research continues to explore new applications of PRP therapy, such as in dermatology for skin rejuvenation and hair loss treatment. By understanding the scientific basis and clinical evidence supporting PRP therapy, healthcare providers can better inform patients about its potential benefits and limitations. Trials have shown that PRP therapy may be safer and more effective than traditional treatments. It has the potential to speed wound healing and tissue regeneration, which is crucial in sports medicine and orthopedic surgery.

CASE STUDIES AND PATIENT TESTIMONIALS

Patient testimonials and case studies offer important perspectives on the practical efficacy of platelet-rich plasma (PRP) therapy. Several patients have experienced notable improvements in their symptoms and overall quality of life after receiving PRP injections; those with chronic joint pain, for instance, frequently report decreased pain and improved mobility following PRP treatments.

Case studies also emphasize customized treatment plans based on the unique responses and conditions of each patient. Patient satisfaction and results are crucial when assessing the practical efficacy of PRP therapy in various medical specialties.

In addition, case studies show how PRP therapy is used in a variety of patient populations, from elderly patients with degenerative joint diseases to athletes with sports injuries. These cases frequently record long-term benefits like continued pain relief and improved joint function, which are important factors to take into account for patients and healthcare providers. By examining patient testimonials and case studies, clinicians can learn a great deal about how to best manage patient expectations and optimize treatment protocols. In the end, these real-world experiences add to the growing body of evidence that supports the clinical use of PRP therapy.

SHORT-TERM VS. LONG-TERM ADVANTAGES

Both patients and healthcare providers should be aware of the differences between the short- and long-term benefits of PRP therapy. Short-term benefits are characterized by the immediate pain relief and inflammation reduction that often follow PRP injections.

These initial effects are often noticeable a few weeks after treatment, giving patients prompt relief from symptoms. Long-term benefits, on the other hand, are characterized by the sustained therapeutic effects of PRP therapy over extended periods. Research suggests that PRP injections can promote tissue regeneration and healing processes that contribute to long-lasting improvements in joint function and mobility.

Furthermore, the duration of PRP therapy's benefits may differ based on the underlying ailment and variables unique to each patient.

For example, people receiving PRP treatments for chronic tendon injuries may gradually improve their tendon strength and flexibility over several months. Long-term research also indicates that PRP therapy may postpone or even eliminate the need for surgical interventions in specific orthopedic conditions. By assessing the benefits of PRP therapy in the short and long term, medical professionals can customize treatment regimens to alleviate immediate symptoms while maximizing results for long-term therapeutic benefits.

COMPARING ALTERNATIVE MEDICAL INTERVENTIONS

When comparing PRP therapy to other treatments, one can gain an important understanding of its relative effectiveness and advantages in clinical practice. Anti-inflammatory medications, physical therapy, and surgical interventions are common treatments for musculoskeletal conditions. PRP therapy, on the other hand, is a non-surgical alternative that uses concentrated platelet injections to stimulate the body's natural healing mechanisms. Studies have indicated that PRP therapy may produce results that are on par with or better than corticosteroid injections for conditions such as osteoarthritis and chronic tendon injuries.

In addition, PRP therapy is widely regarded as safe, minimally invasive, and adverse reaction-free due to its use of the patient's blood components. Surgical interventions, on the other hand, entail inherent risks, including infection, extended recovery times, and potential complications.

Healthcare providers can recommend customized treatment plans that are in line with patient preferences and clinical objectives by comparing the pros and cons of PRP therapy against alternative treatments. These comparative studies further enhance our understanding of PRP therapy's place in contemporary medical practice by highlighting its potential as a viable treatment option across a range of healthcare specialties.

TAKING CARE OF COMMON MISCONCEPTIONS

To promote informed decision-making among patients and healthcare providers, it is imperative to address common misconceptions regarding PRP therapy. Firstly, there is a common misconception that PRP injections provide immediate or miraculous results. Although some patients may experience immediate symptom relief, PRP therapy typically has therapeutic effects that develop gradually as the body goes through its natural healing processes. Secondly, there is a misconception regarding treatment outcomes. Individual responses to PRP therapy can vary depending on factors like age, general health, and the severity of the condition being treated.

Furthermore, a great deal of clinical research and regulatory oversight has been conducted to address concerns regarding the safety and effectiveness of PRP therapy. Research has consistently shown that PRP therapy is safe when administered by qualified professionals using sterile techniques.

In addition, myths regarding PRP therapy's cost-effectiveness in comparison to other treatments should take into account the potential long-term savings from lower healthcare utilization and better patient outcomes. As a result, patients will feel more empowered and transparent when healthcare providers recommend PRP therapy as a viable treatment option.

CHAPTER SEVEN

SECURITY AND POSSIBLE ADVERSE REACTIONS

TYPICAL SIDE EFFECTS FOLLOWING PRP THERAPY

Beginners should be aware that although platelet-rich plasma (PRP) therapy is generally safe, it can have common side effects, such as mild pain, swelling, and bruising at the injection site. These reactions are normal and usually go away in a few days as the body absorbs the PRP and starts the healing process. It is important to let patients know about these potential side effects in advance to manage expectations and make sure they know what to expect after treatment.

Furthermore, some patients may feel warm or hot where the injection was made; this is a normal reaction as the platelets promote healing. To minimize discomfort and guarantee the best possible recovery, it is important for novice PRP therapists to closely monitor their patients following treatment and to provide them with post-care instructions. By educating patients about these typical side effects, practitioners can improve patient satisfaction and lower anxiety related to the course of treatment.

In summary, a proactive approach to patient education about the typical side effects of platelet-rich plasma (PRP) therapy is essential to delivering all-encompassing care. Practitioners can empower patients to identify normal post-treatment reactions and allay concerns by explaining the possibility of mild pain, swelling, bruising, and warmth at the injection site.

HANDLING PAIN AND UNCOMFORT

While mild pain and soreness at the injection site are common, practitioners can employ several strategies to effectively manage these symptoms. One such strategy is to encourage patients to apply ice packs intermittently in the hours following treatment, which can help reduce swelling and numb the area, providing immediate relief.

Managing discomfort and pain following PRP therapy is crucial for ensuring patient comfort and satisfaction.

In addition, prescribing over-the-counter analgesics like acetaminophen or ibuprofen, if appropriate for the patient, can help reduce pain even more. In addition, novices in PRP therapy should instruct patients on how to take these drugs correctly and caution them against aspirin, which can increase the risk of bleeding.

Patients should also be advised to refrain from heavy lifting or strenuous activities for a few days following their procedure to prevent pain from getting worse and to encourage the best possible healing process.

To sum up, ice therapy, pain medication, and activity restriction are all important components of a multimodal approach to managing pain and discomfort following PRP therapy. Practitioners who provide patients with clear instructions and support can improve patient comfort and speed up the healing process. Proactive management also lowers patient anxiety and increases patient satisfaction with PRP therapy results.

COMPLICATIONS AND ALLERGIC REACTIONS

It is rare, but allergic reactions and complications can happen after PRP therapy, so practitioners need to be aware of this and ready for it. Allergic reactions can cause swelling, redness, or itching outside the injection site, which means the patient is allergic to materials used in the procedure or to something in the PRP. Practitioners should keep an eye out for these symptoms as soon as the patient gets them.

More severe cases can cause patients to feel lightheaded, have trouble breathing, or have a fast heartbeat, which is an indication of an anaphylactic reaction that needs to be treated right away. To handle these uncommon but serious complications as soon as they arise, practitioners must have emergency protocols in place that include access to epinephrine and emergency services. Other critical components of safe PRP therapy practice include informing patients about these potential risks and obtaining their informed consent before treatment.

In conclusion, even though allergic reactions and complications are rare, healthcare professionals need to be ready to identify and handle them when they arise. By teaching patients about possible allergic reaction symptoms and setting up emergency procedures, novices can administer safe and responsible care during PRP therapy. This proactive approach not only improves patient safety but also fosters patient confidence in the therapeutic process.

REDUCING HAZARDS THROUGH APPROPRIATE PLANNING

Before beginning treatment, novices should perform a thorough medical assessment of patients to identify any underlying conditions or medications that may increase the risk of complications. This evaluation ensures that PRP therapy is appropriate and safe for the specific patient. Adhering to best practices is the first step in minimizing the risks associated with PRP therapy.

In addition, using sterile equipment and keeping a clean environment are crucial steps in preventing contamination and promoting patient safety. Beginners should make sure they have received the necessary training and certification in PRP therapy techniques to perform the procedure competently and confidently.

Practitioners must adhere to strict aseptic techniques during PRP preparation and administration to minimize the risk of infection.

Let's sum up by saying that reducing risks during PRP therapy necessitates careful planning, which includes patient evaluation, adhering to aseptic protocols, and mastering techniques. Practitioners who prioritize safety measures and professional development can minimize potential complications and offer the best care possible to patients undergoing PRP therapy.

This dedication to safety not only improves treatment outcomes but also fosters patient trust and satisfaction.

WHEN TO GET MEDICAL HELP

Patients should be instructed to closely monitor their symptoms after treatment and to contact their healthcare provider immediately if they experience severe pain, persistent swelling, or signs of infection such as redness, warmth, or drainage at the injection site.

Knowing when to seek medical attention after PRP therapy is crucial for ensuring timely intervention and addressing potential complications.

In addition, practitioners should advise patients to seek medical attention if they experience systemic symptoms, such as fever, chills, nausea, or vomiting, as these could be signs of a more serious reaction or infection. During the pre-treatment consultation, practitioners should educate patients about these warning signs and provide clear instructions on how to contact emergency services or come to the clinic for evaluation.

Patient safety and well-being must identify the warning signs that should prompt medical attention following PRP therapy. Practitioners can also improve patient safety by proactively promoting proactive healthcare-seeking behavior and ensuring prompt intervention when necessary by educating patients about potential complications and emergency procedures.

CHAPTER EIGHT

COMBINING PRP THERAPY WITH OTHER INTERVENTIONS

PRP AND PHYSICAL THERAPY IN COMBINATION

For a variety of musculoskeletal conditions, the use of Platelet-Rich Plasma (PRP) therapy in conjunction with physical therapy has demonstrated encouraging outcomes. The goal of PRP and physical therapy integration is to optimize recovery and improve outcomes through the utilization of targeted rehabilitation exercises and the regenerative properties of PRP.

Physical therapy sessions are designed to support the healing process after PRP administration. Typically, PRP injections are strategically given into the affected area under medical supervision. These injections deliver concentrated growth factors derived from the patient's blood, stimulating tissue repair and reducing inflammation.

Patients benefit from a comprehensive approach that addresses both the structural repair facilitated by PRP and the functional rehabilitation guided by physical therapy professionals when physical therapists collaborate closely with healthcare providers to create customized exercise regimens that support each patient's unique needs. These exercises are designed to strengthen muscles, improve flexibility, and restore functionality to the injured or degenerated tissues.

ADJUNCTIVE UTILIZATION IN SURGICAL OPERATIONS

Platelet-rich plasma (PRP) therapy is frequently used to supplement surgical interventions in orthopedics, sports medicine, and other surgical specialties. Its potential to optimize healing and post-operative recovery has drawn attention to the supplementary use of PRP therapy in surgical operations.

PRP is a concentrated dose of growth factors that promote tissue regeneration and reduce inflammation, which may speed healing and minimize complications. It can be injected into the surrounding tissues or applied directly to the surgical site during procedures.

Medical professionals work together to decide how best to use platelet-rich plasma (PRP) in conjunction with surgical techniques. Based on surgical goals and patient-specific factors, the decision to use PRP as an adjunct therapy is made.

The goal of combining PRP with surgical procedures is to improve patient satisfaction, reduce recovery times, and improve overall outcomes.

SUPPLEMENTAL TREATMENTS FOR BETTER OUTCOMES

To improve treatment outcomes for a range of medical diseases, alternative therapies, such as acupuncture, chiropractic adjustments, and herbal medicine, are frequently used in conjunction with platelet-rich plasma (PRP) therapy.

A holistic approach that takes into account the synergistic benefits of combining various treatment modalities guides the integration of PRP with complementary therapies. For instance, PRP injections may be used in conjunction with acupuncture to support the body's natural healing processes and promote circulation.

By combining PRP with complementary therapies, healthcare teams hope to maximize treatment efficacy, enhance patient well-being, and support all-encompassing healing strategies. Healthcare providers work in tandem with practitioners of complementary therapies to create integrated treatment plans customized to meet the unique needs of each patient.

MULTIDISCIPLINARY METHODS IN MEDICAL ENVIRONMENTS

To address complex medical conditions and improve patient outcomes, multidisciplinary approaches involving Platelet-Rich Plasma (PRP) therapy are becoming more and more common in healthcare settings. These approaches bring together specialists from various disciplines, such as orthopedics, dermatology, and pain management, to collaborate on treatment strategies.

In real practice, a multidisciplinary team of healthcare professionals works together to evaluate patient needs and decide when PRP therapy is best used. This collaborative decision-making process guarantees that PRP is incorporated into a thorough treatment plan that takes into account the particularities of each patient's condition.

Multidisciplinary approaches seek to offer comprehensive care by utilizing the knowledge and skills of various medical professionals. PRP therapy is one type of evidence-based treatment that can be combined with other forms of treatment through this integrated approach, which aims to maximize benefits, minimize risks, and support patient-centered care in various healthcare settings.

WORKING TOGETHER TO MAKE DECISIONS WITH HEALTHCARE PROVIDERS

In the case of Platelet-Rich Plasma (PRP) therapy, close collaboration between healthcare providers is necessary to ensure the best possible treatment outcomes and patient satisfaction. PRP therapy suitability is determined by clinical indications, patient preferences, and treatment goals.

Healthcare providers discuss the potential benefits and risks of PRP therapy, taking into account factors such as the severity of the condition, previous treatment outcomes, and patient expectations. In practice, collaborative decision-making starts with a thorough assessment of the patient's medical history, diagnostic findings, and treatment options.

By giving patients information about PRP therapy and other treatments, shared decision-making enables patients to take an active role in their healthcare journey. This cooperative approach builds treatment adherence, fosters trust, and supports patient-centered care that is in line with their values and preferences.

Healthcare professionals work to provide comprehensive care that incorporates PRP therapy into a larger treatment plan intended to maximize outcomes and enhance patients' quality of life by participating in collaborative decision-making.

CHAPTER NINE

RECOVERY AND REHABILITATION FOLLOWING PROCEDURE

TIMETABLE FOR RECUPERATION AND EXPECTATIONS

It is important to know the recovery schedule and what to anticipate following Platelet-Rich Plasma (PRP) therapy to manage expectations and facilitate a seamless healing process. To allow the PRP injections to take effect, the first phase of recovery usually entails immediate rest and minimal physical activity. Mild discomfort or soreness at the injection site is common during the first few days following the procedure and can be treated with ice packs and over-the-counter pain relievers as directed by your healthcare provider.

Depending on the condition being treated, as the days go into the first week, you might experience gradual improvements in your symptoms. For some conditions, like tendon injuries or joint pain, you might experience some initial relief within the first week to ten days. However, it's important to realize that PRP therapy stimulates the body's natural healing processes, so full recovery frequently takes several weeks to months. Throughout this time, follow-up appointments with your healthcare provider are essential to monitor progress and make any necessary adjustments to the treatment plan.

You may maximize the benefits of PRP therapy and encourage a quicker and more efficient recovery by following your healthcare provider's instructions about activity levels, medication, and follow-up care during the recovery timeline.

LIMITATIONS ON PHYSICAL ACTIVITY

To support healing and optimize treatment outcomes, post-PRP guidelines often include restrictions on physical activity for some time. Patients are typically advised to rest and refrain from physically demanding activities that may put a strain on the treated area.

This period of reduced physical activity allows the PRP injections to settle and initiate healing without interference.

Light walking is generally encouraged in the initial days after PRP therapy to help with circulation and recovery; however, heavy lifting, vigorous exercise, or repetitive motions that could put stress on the injected area should be avoided; your healthcare provider will provide specific recommendations based on your condition and the location of the PRP injections.

Your healthcare provider may gradually introduce more exercises and activities specific to your rehabilitation needs as you move through the recovery timeline.

EXERCISES AND METHODS FOR REHABILITATION

Rehabilitation exercises, which are usually introduced gradually, starting with gentle movements and working up to more challenging activities as healing progresses, are essential for optimizing the benefits of PRP therapy by strengthening muscles, increasing flexibility, and restoring function to the treated area.

Rehabilitation exercises may concentrate on a range of motion exercises, stretching, and targeted strengthening exercises that target the affected area depending on the condition being treated. For instance, eccentric strengthening exercises that are intended to rebuild tendon strength and resilience may be included in the exercises if PRP therapy is used to treat a tendon injury.

To get the most out of PRP therapy and reduce the chance of complications or re-injury, you must perform rehabilitation exercises under the supervision of a licensed healthcare professional.

DIETARY GUIDELINES FOR THE BEST POSSIBLE RECOVERY

A diet rich in lean proteins, fruits, vegetables, and whole grains provides the vitamins, minerals, and antioxidants required for cellular repair and immune function. Optimizing your diet can dramatically accelerate the healing process after PRP therapy by providing vital nutrients that support tissue repair and regeneration.

Because it offers the building blocks for collagen creation and tissue regeneration, protein is very important for tissue healing. You may assist the healing process by including sources of lean protein in your diet, such as fish, poultry, beans, and tofu.

Items high in omega-3 fatty acids, zinc, and vitamin C can help aid in healing and reduce inflammation. Nuts, seeds, citrus fruits, berries, and fatty fish (like salmon) are great items to include in your diet after PRP therapy.

Another crucial component of recovery is hydration; drinking enough water promotes healthy circulation, nutrition delivery to tissues, and general healing; excessive alcohol and sugary drink consumption might compromise the immune system and healing processes.

TRACKING DEVELOPMENT AND MODIFYING THERAPY REGIMENS

After PRP therapy, you should schedule routine follow-up appointments with your physician to monitor your healing process, make any necessary plan adjustments, and guarantee the best possible results. Your physician will examine your symptoms, range of motion, strength, and general function of the treated area.

Your healthcare provider may suggest changes to your rehabilitation program or additional PRP injections to enhance results if your initial progress is slower than expected. Similarly, adjustments to rehabilitation exercises, activity levels, or additional treatments may be suggested based on your progress to support ongoing healing and recovery.

Maintaining open lines of communication with your healthcare provider regarding your recovery experience and any concerns you may have is crucial to optimizing your treatment outcomes.

CHAPTER TEN

EXPENSES, COVERAGE, AND LAWFUL ASPECTS

FACTORS AFFECTING PRP THERAPY COSTS

Patients should be aware of the following costs associated with Platelet-Rich Plasma (PRP) therapy: first, there is the initial consultation with a healthcare provider, during which the patient's suitability for PRP therapy is evaluated based on their medical history and particular condition; second, there are costs associated with the procedure itself, which vary depending on the area of treatment and degree of complexity; third, there may be additional costs associated with processing the blood sample to extract platelets and preparing the PRP injection; and fourth, some clinics charge for follow-up visits to check on patients' progress after treatment.

Patients should ask about the entire cost breakdown at the initial consultation to manage these costs effectively.

It is important to know what each cost component covers and whether there are any hidden fees. Payment plans and financing options are offered by many healthcare providers to help patients manage expenses over time. Additionally, comparing the pricing structures of various clinics can shed light on cost variations and help patients make an informed decision about where to undergo PRP therapy.

By discussing costs up front and looking into payment options, patients can approach PRP therapy with confidence, focusing on achieving their health goals without undue financial stress. Patients who are aware of the financial implications of PRP therapy can plan their budget accordingly and avoid unexpected financial burdens.

OPTIONS FOR INSURANCE COVERAGE AND REIMBURSEMENT

Insurance coverage for PRP therapy varies greatly depending on the insurance company and the particular policy.

Generally speaking, if PRP therapy is deemed experimental or investigational, it may not be covered by insurance for certain medical conditions. On the other hand, some insurance plans may cover PRP therapy for certain indications, such as osteoarthritis or chronic tendon injuries, particularly when conservative treatments have failed.

If insurance does not cover PRP therapy, patients can look into other financing options like health savings accounts (HSAs) or flexible spending accounts (FSAs), which can be used to pay for qualified medical expenses. Before receiving PRP therapy, patients should speak with their insurance provider to learn about coverage details and potential out-of-pocket costs. It's also important to get pre-authorization if necessary and to understand any deductible or co-payment obligations.

Options for PRP therapy reimbursement can also differ based on medical professionals and facilities; some offer self-pay discounts or package deals for several treatment sessions, which can lower overall costs; patients should carefully consider all available options for reimbursement to make an educated decision about pursuing PRP therapy and managing related costs.

REGULATIONS AND LAWS

Healthcare providers who offer PRP therapy must abide by legal and regulatory guidelines to ensure patient safety and treatment efficacy. These guidelines may include standards for handling blood products, protocols for patient monitoring and follow-up care, and licensing requirements for performing the procedure. Regulatory bodies and professional organizations also provide guidelines to healthcare providers to ensure PRP therapy is administered safely and ethically.

Before giving informed consent, patients have the right to know the risks, benefits, and alternatives of PRP therapy. They should also find out the credentials and qualifications of healthcare providers who offer PRP therapy to make sure they are properly trained and licensed. Receiving treatment in a facility that complies with regulatory standards and maintains proper documentation of procedures and outcomes is also important.

Patients can increase their chances of achieving positive treatment outcomes while minimizing potential risks by selecting reputable healthcare providers and facilities that prioritize patient safety and compliance with regulations. Patients can make informed decisions about their healthcare by being aware of the legal and regulatory framework surrounding PRP therapy.

RIGHTS OF THE PATIENT AND INFORMED CONSENT

Patients undergoing PRP therapy have the right to clear and comprehensive information about the procedure, including its purpose, potential benefits, risks, and alternative treatments. Healthcare providers must also ensure that patients understand the nature of PRP therapy and provide an opportunity for patients to express concerns and ask questions. In PRP therapy, patient rights include the right to privacy, autonomy, and information throughout the treatment process.

Patients must sign a consent form acknowledging that they have read and understand the risks and benefits of PRP therapy. They must also be informed about any potential side effects, such as temporary discomfort at the injection site or uncommon complications like infection or allergic reaction. Informed consent is a crucial component of PRP therapy.

Patients also have the right to confidentiality and privacy regarding the medical information they provide for PRP therapy. Healthcare providers are required to follow legal and ethical guidelines to protect patient confidentiality and individual privacy rights.

Patients who are aware of their rights and actively participate in the informed consent process can make well-informed decisions about PRP therapy while maintaining the security of their personal and medical information.

BUDGETING AND FINANCIAL PLANNING FOR MEDICAL TREATMENT

Financial planning for PRP therapy entails estimating costs, investigating insurance coverage, and locating possible funding sources or payment options. Patients should begin by requesting a comprehensive cost estimate from their physician that includes consultation fees, procedure costs, and any other costs like lab fees or follow-up visits. It's also important to find out what payment methods the clinic accepts and whether they provide financing options or installment plans to spread costs over time.

Those without insurance coverage for PRP therapy may want to use health savings accounts (HSAs) or flexible spending accounts (FSAs) to cover eligible medical expenses; some healthcare providers also offer self-pay discounts or package deals for multiple treatment sessions, which can help reduce overall costs. For patients with insurance coverage, it's important to understand deductibles, co-payments, and coverage limitations for budgetary purposes.

By investigating all financial factors, such as insurance coverage, reimbursement options, and potential out-of-pocket costs, patients can approach PRP therapy with confidence and focus on achieving optimal health outcomes without financial strain. Developing a financial plan for PRP therapy enables patients to budget effectively and make educated decisions about their healthcare expenses.

CHAPTER ELEVEN
COMMON QUESTIONS AND EXTENSIVE ANSWERS
TAKING CARE OF THE PAIN AND NEEDLES FEAR

Many people who are thinking about getting Platelet-Rich Plasma (PRP) therapy may be worried about needles and possible pain during the procedure. However, it's important to know that even though needles are used to draw blood and inject PRP into the treatment area, there is usually very little discomfort during the process. Topical numbing agents are frequently applied to the skin before the procedure to help minimize any discomfort during the injection process.

In addition, PRP therapy providers are trained to guarantee patient safety and comfort throughout the process; they also use fine-gauge needles for PRP injection and blood collection, which further reduces discomfort; patients can discuss any pain concerns with their provider, who can modify the treatment plan to optimize comfort; and finally, knowing that PRP therapy discomfort is usually mild and transient can allay worries and put patients at ease during the procedure.

CONTROLLING TREATMENT OUTCOME EXPECTATIONS

Setting realistic expectations involves talking about potential outcomes with a healthcare provider who can offer insights based on the patient's particular case and medical history. While PRP has shown promising results in promoting healing and reducing pain, individual responses to treatment can vary. Patients must understand that the outcomes of PRP therapy depend on several factors, including the specific condition being treated, the severity of the condition, and the individual's overall health.

Patients should be ready for the possibility of gradual improvements over time rather than immediate, dramatic changes.

Open communication between patients and healthcare providers ensures that expectations are aligned with the potential benefits and limitations of PRP therapy. This approach helps patients make informed decisions about their treatment journey and enhances satisfaction with the overall outcomes. Some patients may experience noticeable improvements in symptoms and function shortly after treatment; in other cases, multiple sessions may be needed to achieve optimal results.

EXTENDED DURABILITY OF OUTCOMES

One of the most important factors for patients receiving PRP therapy is the sustainability of treatment outcomes over the long term. Although PRP can offer substantial relief and improvement in several conditions, the length of time that results last can vary based on the particular condition treated and each patient's healing response.

Research indicates that PRP may promote tissue regeneration and repair, which may prolong symptom relief and improve functional outcomes in certain cases. However, lifestyle factors like activity level, diet, and general health maintenance can also affect how long results last.

Patients are often advised to adhere to post-treatment care instructions from their healthcare provider to optimize the sustainability of PRP therapy results. These instructions may include recommendations for dietary changes, activity modifications, and possible follow-up treatments.

Scheduling regular follow-up appointments enables healthcare providers to monitor patient progress, address any concerns, and suggest additional PRP sessions as needed. Patients can support the long-term benefits of PRP therapy and improve their overall health outcomes by actively participating in their recovery process and following recommended guidelines.

NUMBER OF PRP THERAPY SESSIONS PER MONTH

Patients who are thinking about PRP therapy should know how often these sessions should be scheduled. The number of sessions that should be scheduled can vary depending on the particular condition being treated as well as the response of each patient. PRP therapy frequently entails a series of initial treatments spaced out over several weeks to maximize therapeutic benefits. This allows the body to react to the treatment and effectively start healing processes.

Healthcare providers create individualized treatment schedules based on the patient's condition severity, treatment goals, and response to prior PRP sessions. Patients are encouraged to discuss treatment frequency with their healthcare provider to develop a plan that fits their needs and expectations for recovery. For acute injuries or conditions, patients may benefit from more frequent PRP sessions initially, followed by maintenance treatments as needed. Chronic conditions may require a longer-term treatment plan with periodic PRP sessions to maintain symptom relief and functional improvement.

PATIENT EMPOWERMENT AND EDUCATION

Healthcare providers explain how PRP is prepared from the patient's blood, emphasizing its natural healing properties and safety profile. Patient education plays a crucial role in the success of PRP therapy by empowering individuals to make informed decisions about their health.

Patients can develop confidence and trust in the therapy by learning about the science behind PRP, its potential benefits, and the treatment process.

Furthermore, patient empowerment entails providing resources, such as informational materials and access to medical professionals, to support ongoing communication and decision-making throughout the treatment course.

This collaborative approach fosters a positive patient-provider relationship and enhances overall satisfaction with PRP therapy outcomes. Although potential risks and complications are generally rare, understanding the treatment process and possible outcomes empowers patients to actively participate in their care journey, ask informed questions, and work with healthcare providers to achieve optimal results.